RENAL DIET SMOOTHIE RECIPES

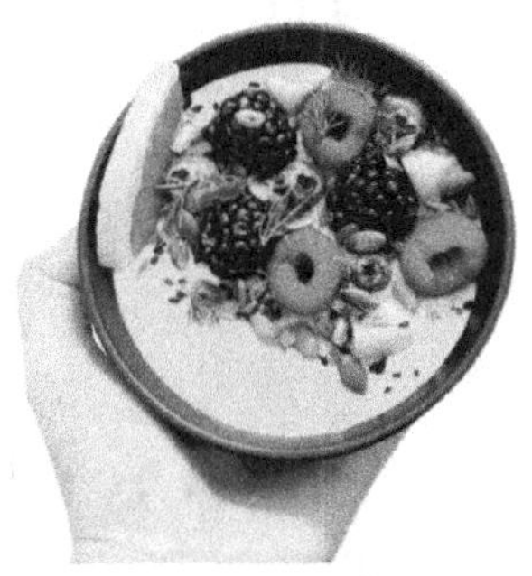

A Delicious Approach To Juicing For Optimum Kidney Health, Prevention and Management of Kidney Problems

Nancy K. Doctor

Copyright © 2023 Nancy K. Doctor

All rights reserved.

OTHER BOOKS WRITTEN BY THE AUTHOR
SCAN THIS ⬆

TABLE OF CONTENTS

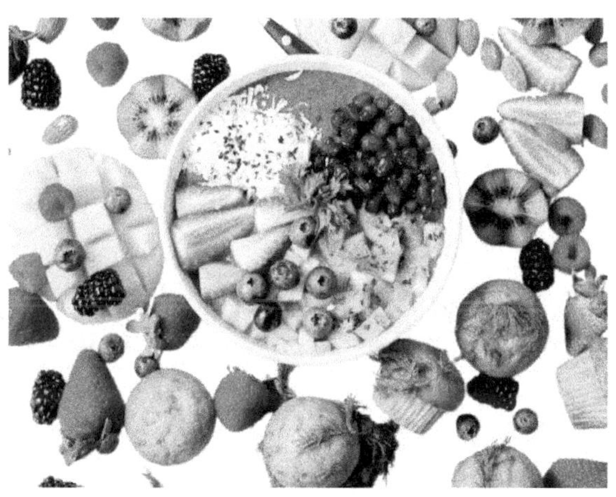

"Nourish your body with delicious smoothies, and watch your kidney health bloom. Empower your kidney function with every sip of a renal-friendly smoothie."

INTRODUCTION

Have you ever felt that your kidney disease diagnosis has limited your meal options to bland, unappealing fare?

Do you wish you could eat tasty and healthy meals that promote kidney health without feeling limited or restricted?

These are the same questions Sarah is thinking about. Sarah, a lively 45-year-old lady, has always been committed to leading a healthy lifestyle. Her diagnosis of chronic renal illness, on the other hand, turned her world upside down. She was instructed to adhere to a tight, limited diet, which left her feeling starved and uninspired.

Sarah immediately dove into the pages of "Renal Diet Smoothie Recipes" as her guide, intrigued by the concept of including smoothies into her kidney-friendly diet. A ray of hope appeared when she found a world of delectable and healthful smoothie choices.

Sarah enthusiastically embraced the smoothie recipes and began adding them to her regular regimen. She savored the energizing berry combinations, energizing tropical concoctions, and creamy protein-packed smoothies. She had a restored feeling of vigor and well-being as she cherished each sip.

Sarah's life changed with each smoothie she drank. Her limited diet was no longer a strain; it had evolved into a gastronomic adventure. She found new flavors and textures while fueling her body and satisfying her taste senses.

You may also embark on a culinary trip to renal health with "Renal Diet Smoothie Recipes," a one-stop guide to tasty and nutritious smoothies that promote kidney function and general well-being. Say goodbye to dull, restrictive meals and hello to a world of taste and nutrients with our specifically prepared recipes, which are tailored to the unique needs of people with renal disease.

This thorough resource contains a treasure trove of smoothie recipes that are not only kidney-friendly but also delicious. Our smoothies are high in vitamins, minerals, and antioxidants, which help kidney function and enhance overall wellness.

You'll be whipping up kidney-friendly smoothies in no time, bringing a touch of fun to your daily routine while feeding your health, thanks to clear directions and simple advice. So grab your blender and get ready to go on a smoothie adventure that will change the way you think about kidney-conscious eating.

CHAPTER 1
KIDNEY-FRIENDLY FRUIT & FOOD

Our kidneys, the hidden heroes of our bodies, serve an important function in filtering waste from our blood and preserving general health. When these vital organs are harmed, it is critical to adopt dietary changes to support their function and avoid future damage. A kidney-friendly diet emphasizes nutrient-rich meals while reducing those that might impose pressure on the kidneys, ensuring that these critical organs work properly.

Fruits and Vegetables' Place in a Kidney-Friendly Diet

Fruits and vegetables are not only tasty complements to our meals; they are also high in nutrients that promote kidney function. These nutrient-dense meals include important vitamins, minerals, and antioxidants that protect cells from harm and may help lower the risk of renal disease.

Fruits That Are Good For Your Kidneys

A variety of kidney-friendly fruits in your diet can give you a plethora of health advantages. Here are some of the best options for including in your meals:

*1. **Berries:*** Berries, which include blueberries, strawberries, raspberries, and cranberries, are high in antioxidants, which protect cells from harm and may help lower the risk of kidney disease. Their high fiber content helps intestinal health as well.

*2. **Apples:*** Apples are versatile and fiber-rich, making them an excellent complement to a kidney-friendly diet. They are high in potassium, vitamin C, and fiber, all of which are helpful for kidney function. They can be eaten as a refreshing snack, added to salads, or baked into pies or muffins.

*3. **Grapes:*** Resveratrol, an antioxidant with anti-inflammatory qualities that may help preserve the kidneys, is found in grapes, particularly red grapes. Eat them raw as a snack or add them to salads or desserts.

*4. **Watermelon:*** Watermelon is a delicious and hydrating fruit that is low in potassium and phosphorus, making it a good choice for persons who have renal illness. Its high water content aids in fluid balance and the removal of pollutants.

*5. **Pears*** are a pleasant and delicious fruit that is high in fiber and potassium. They're also low in phosphorus, so they're a good choice for kidney-friendly diets. Serve them sliced, cooked, or blended into smoothies.

Vegetables for Kidneys

Vegetables are an essential component of a diet that is beneficial for kidney health. They include a variety of vitamins, minerals, and fiber, all of which improve kidney function and general health. Here are some of the best kidney-friendly veggies to incorporate into your diet:

1. Cauliflower: This versatile vegetable may be prepared in a variety of ways, including roasting, steaming, or mashing. It has a low potassium and phosphorus content, making it a good choice for kidney-friendly diets. Cauliflower may be used in soups, stews, or rice alternatives.

2. Cabbage is a cruciferous vegetable that is high in fiber and vitamin C. It is also low in potassium and phosphorus, making it a good choice for people with renal problems. Enjoy raw cabbage in salads, cooked cabbage, or fermented cabbage as sauerkraut.

3. Bell peppers: Bell peppers, especially the red and yellow types, are high in vitamin C and antioxidants. They also have a low potassium and phosphorus content. Grill, roast, or stuff bell peppers with quinoa or other kidney-friendly contents.

4. *Cucumbers:* Cucumbers are refreshing and hydrating, and they are low in potassium and phosphorus. They are also a rich source of potassium, which is necessary for fluid equilibrium. Cucumbers may be used in salads, sandwiches, or as a refreshing snack.

5. *Celery* is a low-calorie vegetable that is high in fiber and potassium. It's also low in phosphorus, making it ideal for kidney-friendly diets. Celery stalks may be eaten with hummus, added to soups or stews, or mixed into salads for a crisp crunch.

General Kidney-Friendly Diet Advice

Aside from selecting kidney-friendly fruits and vegetables, here are some basic guidelines for eating a kidney-friendly diet:

1. *Limit Sodium Consumption:* Aim for fewer than 2,300 milligrams of sodium per day, preferably less than 1,500 milligrams per day. When possible, read food labels carefully and seek low-sodium products.

2. *Control Your Potassium Intake:* Consult your doctor to calculate your daily potassium requirements. Keep an eye on the potassium amount of your meal choices and make changes as required.

3. Phosphorus consumption should be monitored: Aim for fewer than 1,000 mg of phosphorus per day. Limit processed meals and dairy products while eating low-phosphorus protein sources such as lean meats, fish, and eggs.

4. Protein Intake Should Be Adjusted: Your recommended daily protein intake may differ based on your renal function. Consult your doctor for advice on the proper quantity of protein for your specific needs.

5. Follow your doctor's recommendations for fluid consumption, which may vary depending on your specific needs.

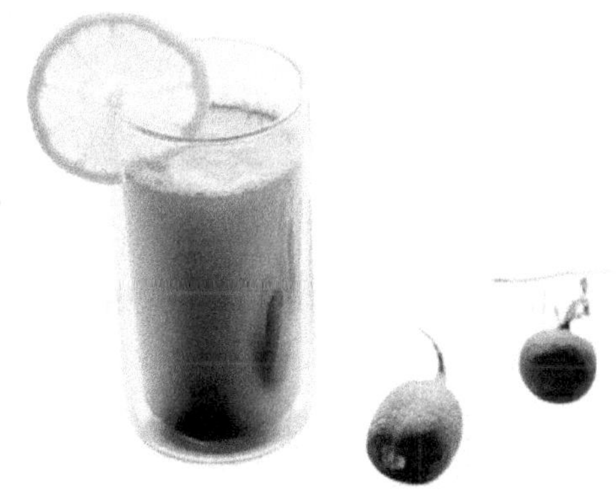

CHAPTER 2
DIETARY MODIFICATIONS FOR KIDNEY DISEASE

The kidneys, our body's relentless filters, play an important part in general health maintenance by eliminating waste materials and excess fluids from the blood. When kidney function degrades, it can develop into chronic kidney disease (CKD), a degenerative disorder that can impact many aspects of health if left untreated.

While there is no treatment for CKD, dietary changes can slow the disease's progression and help people manage their symptoms and retain a decent quality of life. A renal-friendly diet that is well-planned can help delay the deterioration of kidney function, avoid future issues, and enhance general well-being.

The Fundamentals of a Kidney-Friendly Diet

A kidney-friendly diet emphasizes nutrient-rich meals while avoiding those that might strain the kidneys, such as those heavy in salt, potassium, phosphorus, and protein. Depending on the stage of CKD and the individual's general health, the particular dietary recommendations for a kidney-friendly diet may differ. However, some broad concepts are as follows:

1. Reducing Sodium Intake: Sodium is important for fluid balance, but too much of it can strain the kidneys and lead to fluid accumulation in the body. Aim for fewer than 2,300 milligrams of salt per day, preferably less than 1,500 mg.

2. Potassium Consumption: Potassium is an important element, but people with CKD may need to limit their consumption to avoid harmful amounts of potassium in the blood. Adults with CKD should consume between 2,000 and 4,000 mg of potassium each day.

3. Managing Phosphorus Intake: Another mineral that can accumulate in the blood of people with CKD is phosphorus. Limiting your phosphorus consumption might help you avoid bone disorders and other health issues. The typical daily phosphorus intake for adults with CKD is 500 to 1,000 milligrams.

4. Protein: is an essential nutrient for many bodily functions, but people with advanced kidney disease may need to limit their protein intake to reduce the strain on their kidneys. Adults with renal illness should consume 0.6 to 0.8 grams of protein per kilogram of body weight daily.

5. *Fluid Management: People* with renal illness may need to limit their fluid consumption to avoid fluid accumulation in the body. Adults with renal illness should drink between 1,500 and 2,000 milliliters of liquids every day.

Options For A Kidney-friendly Diet

A range of renal-friendly meals can deliver important nutrients while also supporting kidney function. Here are some meals that are good for your kidneys:

1. Fruits: *D*ue to their low potassium and phosphorus content, berries, apples, grapes, watermelon, and pears are excellent choices for kidney-friendly diets.

2. Cauliflower, cabbage, bell peppers, cucumbers, and celery are low in potassium and phosphorus, making them ideal for kidney-friendly diets.

3. Protein Sources: A kidney-friendly diet can include lean meats, fish, eggs, low-fat dairy products, and plant-based proteins like beans and lentils in moderation.

4. Olive oil, avocados, and nuts are high in heart-healthy fats and can be included in a kidney-friendly diet in moderation.

5. Whole Grains: Fiber-rich whole grains such as brown rice, quinoa, and whole-wheat bread can be included in a kidney-friendly diet.

Limiting Potassium, Phosphorus, and Sodium-Rich Foods

While some foods are good for your kidneys, others should be limited or avoided because of their high potassium, phosphorus, and sodium content. These are some examples:

1. Processed foods frequently have high levels of sodium, potassium, and phosphorus. Processed meats, canned foods, frozen meals, and salty snacks should be limited or avoided.

2. High-Potassium Fruits and Vegetables: While many fruits and vegetables are beneficial for a kidney-friendly diet, some, such as oranges, bananas, potatoes, and tomatoes, are high in potassium and should be limited or avoided.

3. High-Phosphorus Foods: Dairy products, organ meats, and some nuts and seeds are high in phosphorus. Limiting your intake of these foods can help you manage your blood phosphorus levels.

Why Are Smoothies So Popular?

Smoothies have grown in popularity over the years, with many people turning to these delicious and nutritious concoctions to meet their daily vitamin and mineral requirements. However, they can be much more effective for those who have chronic renal disease or are on dialysis.

Smoothies, in addition to delivering critical nutrients, are generally easier for CKD and dialysis patients to manage than solid diets since portion management is considerably simpler.

Incorporating smoothies into a renal diet has a slew of advantages for those with kidney disease. Smoothies are a quick and easy method to get critical nutrients, fluids, and antioxidants that help kidney function and general health.

1. Nutrient-dense And Easily Digestible

Smoothies are an easy way to incorporate a range of nutrient-dense fruits, vegetables, and kidney-friendly components. They include a high concentration of vitamins, minerals, and fiber, which promote general health and renal function. Smoothies are also simple to digest, making them an excellent choice for people who have a low appetite or digestive concerns.

2. Hydration Assistance

Smoothies are a fantastic method to improve fluid consumption, which is essential for kidney health. Watermelon, cucumbers, and celery are examples of hydrating fruits and vegetables that can assist in satisfying daily fluid requirements.

3. Increased Antioxidant Power

Smoothies are high in antioxidants, which help protect cells from harm and may reduce the risk of kidney disease consequences. Fruits and vegetables high in antioxidants, such as berries, grapes, and bell peppers, are ideal complements to renal smoothies.

4. Delicious And Practical

Smoothies are a tasty and entertaining way to include kidney-friendly foods in your diet. Smoothies that are both nutritious and pleasurable may be made by experimenting with different combinations of fruits, vegetables, and other kidney-friendly components.

5. Meal or Snack Replacement

Smoothies may be a handy and healthful lunch or snack alternative. For breakfast, a smoothie packed with protein powder, berries, and spinach may give a healthy start to the day. As a snack, a refreshing smoothie prepared with watermelon, cucumbers, and lemon can help retain hydration and deliver critical nutrients.

Tips For Creating Renal-Friendly Smoothies

1. Choose kidney-friendly fruits and vegetables: Opt for fruits and vegetables that are low in potassium and phosphorus, such as berries, apples, grapes, melons, pears, cauliflower, cabbage, bell peppers, cucumbers, and celery.

2. Include low-fat protein sources: Add protein powder, Greek yogurt, or tofu to your smoothies for an extra burst of protein, which is crucial for maintaining muscle mass.

3. Monitor portion sizes: Be aware of portion amounts, especially when adding fruits, as some might be higher in potassium. Consult your healthcare physician or certified nutritionist for information on optimal portion amounts.

4. Limit extra sweets: Avoid adding excessive sweeteners to your smoothies. Opt for natural sweeteners like honey or maple syrup in moderation, or consider utilizing artificial sweeteners that are permitted for renal diets.

5. Seek Expert Advice: Collaborate with your healthcare team, including your doctor and a qualified dietitian, to create a tailored renal diet plan that incorporates smoothies. They may assist you in selecting proper foods, monitoring nutritional consumption, and making any modifications.

Tips For Blending

When it comes to preparing kidney-friendly smoothies, components are crucial. Aside from picking low-phosphorus, low-potassium fruits and veggies, try utilizing protein powders as an alternative to milk-based nutrients.

Blending your smoothie with ice can assist in minimizing the quantity of liquid you need, while still getting the proper smoothness. Portion control is also key - aim for one to two servings each day. Finally, remember to keep any surplus smoothies in an air-tight container and consume them within 48 hours.

When it comes to blending, the key is making sure that all ingredients are fully integrated. To achieve the best results, use a high-speed blender or food processor.

When incorporating yogurt substitutes such as almond milk, coconut water, or even Greek yogurt, remember that they have more calories than conventional milk.

Additionally, when creating a smoothie, keep taste combinations in mind at all times. Combining sweet and salty fruits with creamy nut butter (such as peanut butter) can assist in producing an intriguing flavor profile that will not get dull after just one try!

Finally, hydration suggestions should be followed to ensure that your drink has enough liquid so that the consistency isn't too thick - this can simply be achieved by adding some ice cubes or your preferred extra liquid.

Smoothie bowls, which include topping your mix with various combinations of nuts, seeds, and dried fruit for extra texture and nutrients, are another wonderful choice for those who like something heartier.

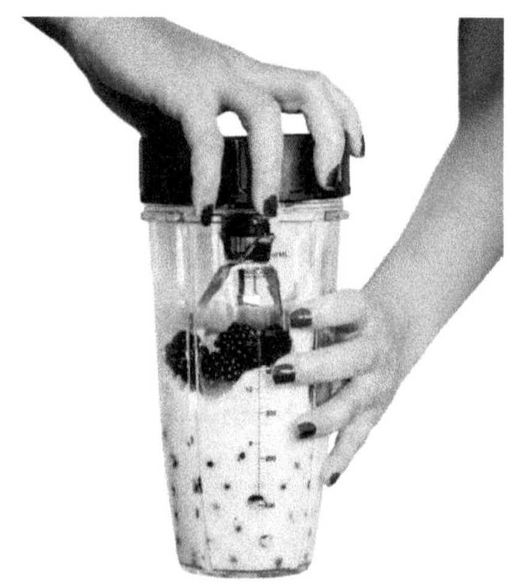

CHAPTER 3
KIDNEY-FRIENDLY SMOOTHIE RECIPES

1. Delightful Triple Berry

Ingredients:
- 1 cup berries
- ½ cup berries
- 12 fresh blackberries
- 2 cups coconut milk or 1 cup almond milk
- 1 cup baby spinach

Preparation:
1. Strawberries, raspberries, blackberries, and a handful of baby spinach are added to the blender.
2. 2 cups coconut milk or almond milk should be added to the mix.
3. Blend until smooth and the desired smoothie texture is achieved.
4. Pour the smoothie into a glass and top with fresh sliced strawberries.

2. Blended Wake-Up Call

Ingredients:
- 1 cup frozen strawberries
- ½ cup frozen mango
- ½ cup pineapple
- 1-quart almond milk

Preparation:
1. Blend in the frozen raspberries, mango, and pineapple.
2. Add in a cup of almond milk and blend until smooth and the ideal smoothie texture is achieved!
3. Serve in a glass, and drink!

3. The Aruba Breeze

Ingredients:
- ½ cup strawberries
- ½ cup pineapple
- 1 mandarin orange, tiny
- 1-quart almond milk
- A spoonful of spinach

Preparation:
1. Blend in the frozen strawberries and pineapple.
2. Peel and cut the orange in half. Blend orange in the blender.

3. Mix with some almond milk and a handful of spinach.
4. Blend until smooth and the desired smoothie texture is achieved!
5. Smoothie should be served in a glass.

4. Smoothie With Berries And Tofu

Ingredients:
- 1 pound fresh strawberries, washed and hulled
- 2 cups fresh blueberries
- 9 ounces silken extra firm tofu
- ½ teaspoon ginger powder
- 2 teaspoons red pepper flakes
- ¼ tsp rum extract
- 1 teaspoon honey
- 1 tsp. lemon juice
- ½ cup of ice

Preparation:
- Put all the ingredients into a blender and blend them together.
- Then, enjoy your drink!

Nutritional info:
- Calories: 136, Carbohydrates: 25.7g, Fiber: 4.2g, Protein: 5.8g, Fat: 2.4g, Sodium: 25.7mg, Potassium: 365.8mg, Calcium: 44.4mg, Phosphorus: 94.8mg

5. Smoothie With Blueberries And Cranberries

Ingredients:
- ½ cup filtered water
- 1 cup blueberries, frozen
- ½ cup fresh or frozen cranberries
- 1 pound red grapes

Instructions:
1. Grapes should be washed.
2. If using fresh cranberries, wash them beforehand.
3. Fill your blender jar halfway with everything, blend for 45-60 seconds, or until smooth

6. Smoothie With Unsweetened Berries And Tofu

Ingredients:
- ¼ cup cranberry juice (mixed)
- ⅓ cup silken tofu, firm
- ½ cup unsweetened frozen raspberries
- ½ cup unsweetened frozen blueberries
- 1 tsp. vanilla extract

Preparation:
1. Pour the juice into a blender and add the remaining ingredients.
2. Blend until completely smooth.
3. Serve immediately and enjoy!

Nutritional info:
- Calories 188, Fat 3g, Carbohydrates 28g, Sodium 6mg, Protein 8g, Potassium 163mg, Phosphorus 30mg, Calcium 165mg.

7. Protein Smoothie for Kidney Health

Ingredients:
- 1 cup frozen cranberries (150g)
- 2 ounces (80g) silken tofu
- 1 cup/220ml nondairy milk
- 1 tiny banana, sliced and frozen.
- 1 tablespoon raw honey or maple syrup (vegan)

Preparation:
1. Mix all the ingredients in a blender until they are completely blended.
2. Taste and adjust the sweetness to your preference if necessary.
3. Serve!

Nutritional info:

- Sugar content: 33.2g, Fiber content: 6.3g, Calories: 278kcal, Fat content: 2.2g, Protein content: 11.7g, Carbohydrate content: 38.2g

8. Smoothie with Cranberries and Pineapple

Ingredients:
- Cranberries juice (34 cup)
- ½ cup fresh or frozen cranberries
- 1 cup pineapple chunks, frozen
- ½ apple

Instructions:
1. If you're using fresh cranberries, wash them beforehand.
2. The apple should be washed, cored, and chopped.
3. Fill your blender jar halfway with everything.
4. Blend the mix for 30 to 45 seconds, or until a homogeneous consistency is achieved.

9. Blend of Daydreaming

Ingredients:
- 1 cup strawberries, frozen
- ½ cup frozen peaches
- 1 cup unsweetened yogurt

- ½ cup coconut water
- 1 fresh strawberry for decoration

Preparation:
1. Blend in the frozen strawberries and peaches.
2. 1 cup plain yogurt and ½ cup coconut water should be added to your mix.
3. Blend until smooth and the desired smoothie texture is achieved!
4. Serve in a glass and garnish with additional fresh herbs or sliced strawberries.

10. Smoothie with Peaches and Raspberries

Ingredients:
- 1 cup raspberries, frozen
- 1 medium pitted and sliced peach
- 1 pound tofu
- 1 tablespoon honey (or sweetener of choice, such as stevia or Splenda)
- 1 cup unsweetened almond milk

Preparation:
- In a blender, combine all of the ingredients and mix until smooth.

Nutritional info:

- Calories: 129 kilocalories, Protein: 6.3g, Carbohydrates: 23g, Fibre: 4.8g, Total Fat: 3.2g, Sodium: 53 mg, Phosphorus: 72mg, Potassium: 261mg

11. Smoothie With Peaches

Ingredients:
- ⅓ cup plain Greek yogurt
- a half-cup almond milk
- 1 frozen peach cup
- 1 tablespoon honey
- 4 cubes of ice

Preparation:
1. Blend Greek yogurt, almond milk, frozen peaches, honey, and ice cubes in a blender.
2. Blend until desired consistency is reached.
3. Pour into a cup and serve!

Nutritional info:
- Calories: 140, Sodium: 80mg, Potassium: 235mg, Phosphorus: 65mg, Carbohydrates: 20g, Protein: 4g.

12. Smoothie with Peaches and High-Protein Fruit

Ingredients:
- ½ cup of ice

- 2 tbsp. Just Whites® (egg white powder)
- ¾ cup peaches, fresh
- 1 teaspoon sugar

Preparation:

1. Blend the peaches in a blender until smooth.
2. Blend in all of the remaining ingredients until smooth.

Tips:

- Just Whites® are powdered egg whites that may be found in the baking area of your local grocery store. Because the product has been pasteurized, it is safe to consume without cooking.
- If using frozen peaches, replace the ice with 1/4 cup water.
- To taste, adjust the sugar or substitute a low-calorie sweetener.

Nutritional information:

- 132 calories, 10g protein, 24g carbohydrates, 0g fat, 154mg sodium, 353mg potassium, 36mg phosphorus, 9mg calcium, and 1.9g fiber

13. Smoothie With Strawberries And Cheesecake

Ingredients:

- 1 cup rice milk, unsweetened

- 1 cup hulled strawberries
- 2 tablespoons room temperature cream cheese
- ½ teaspoon of honey
- A tsp vanilla extract
- 3–5 ice cubes

Instructions:

- Combine the rice milk, strawberries, cream cheese, honey, vanilla, and ice cubes in a blender. Serve after processing until smooth.

Tips:

- Make your cheesecake smoothie by replacing the strawberries with your favorite fruit. This treat works well with blackberries, blueberries, and raspberries.

Nutritional info:

- Calories: 109, Cholesterol: 16mg, Protein: 1g, Sodium: 85mg, Calcium: 60mg, Phosphate: 45mg, Potassium: 139mg

14. Strawberry Fruit Smoothie with High Protein

Ingredients:

- 1 cup of fresh strawberries
- ½ cup pasteurized liquid egg whites
- ½ cup of ice
- 1 teaspoon sugar

Preparation:
1. Blend strawberries till smooth in a blender.
2. Blend in all of the remaining ingredients until smooth.

Tips:
- If using frozen fruit, use ¼ cup water instead of ½ cup ice.
- To taste, add more sugar or a low-calorie sweetener.

Nutritional information:
- 156 calories, 14g protein, 25g carbohydrates, 0g fat, 215mg sodium, 400mg potassium, 49mg phosphorus, 29mg calcium, 2.5g fiber

15. Healthy Cucumber Smoothie

Ingredients:
- 1 medium cucumber (peeled and sliced)
- 1 cup blueberries, fresh or frozen
- 1 cup coconut water (or your favorite nut milk or filtered water)
- 1 to 2 tablespoons ground flax or chia seeds
- 1 tsp cinnamon
- 1 tsp fresh lime juice
- 1 cup of ice
- To taste (Stevia)

Preparation:

1. Place all of the ingredients in the Vitamix container in the order stated and close the lid.
2. Choose speed 1, turn on the machine, and quickly increase to the maximum speed.
3. If necessary, use a tamper to effectively push the ingredients into the blades while processing.
4. Blend for 45-60 seconds, or until you get the desired consistency.
5. Stop the machine and begin serving.

16. Yummy Strawberry-Banana Blend

Ingredients:
- ½ cup (frozen) strawberries
- 1 banana, tiny
- 4 ounces plain 2% yogurt
- 1 teaspoon peanut butter
- 1 cup almond milk, unsweetened
- 1 tablespoon vanilla extract

Preparation:
1. Blend the frozen strawberries and cut bananas in a blender.
2. Mix in the Greek yogurt, a spoonful of peanut butter, a cup of almond milk (or your

preferred milk), and a teaspoon of vanilla essence.

3. Blend until smooth and the ideal smoothie texture is achieved!
4. Serve the smoothie in a glass and enjoy!

Nutritional information:

- 289mg sodium, 12.9g protein, 37mg potassium, 267mg phosphorus, 554mg calcium, 310 calories, 11.2g fat, 42g carbohydrates

17. Smoothie with Low Potassium

Ingredients:

- 1 cup berries, fresh
- 1 frozen pineapple cup
- a third of a cup of ice
- 1-quart rice milk
- 2 scoops of protein powder recommended by a doctor
- 2 to 3 tbsp hemp hearts or chia seeds

Instructions:

- Blend all of the ingredients in a blender. To reach the correct consistency, add additional ice or liquid.

Nutritional info:

- Calories: 265.76kcal, Carbohydrates: 36.91g, Protein: 14.27g, Fat: 8.68g,

Saturated Fat: 0.77g, Potassium: 96.28mg, Sugar: 15.81g, Calcium: 253.23mg.

18. Low Potassium Recipe

Ingredients:
- ½ cup mixed frozen berries or frozen blueberries
- 4 tbsp Whipped Nondairy Topping
- 1 tablespoon Whey Protein Powder
- ¼ cup water (more water as needed)
- Optional: Crystal Light Raspberry Peach

Instructions:
1. Blend all of the ingredients for 45-60 seconds.
2. Add water as needed to get the desired consistency based on your fluid requirements or constraints, as well as your tastes.

19. Gut Smoothie For Kidneys

Ingredients:
- ½ banana
- 1 cup blueberries, frozen
- 1 oz. walnuts
- 1 pound cashew yogurt

Preparation:

1. In a blender, combine all of the ingredients and mix until smooth.
2. Depending on the consistency you want, add additional water/ice. Enjoy!

Nutritional info:

- 525 calories, 14gm protein, 615mg potassium, 10 mg sodium, 11gm fiber

20. Smoothie with Berries for Breakfast

Ingredients:

- 1 medium peeled and sliced cucumber
- ½ cup blueberries, fresh
- ½ cup ripe strawberries
- ½ cup rice milk, unsweetened
- To taste (optional) stevia
- Wheat grass or mint are optional add-ins for added nutrition!

Preparation:

- Simply combine all of the ingredients in a blender, blend until smooth, and enjoy!

Tips:

- Fill your blender no more than two-thirds full. If your blender is having trouble crushing all of the ingredients, add some more rice milk or water!

Nutritional information:

- 115 calories roughly, 150mg of potassium

21. Quinoa with Banana

Ingredients:
- 1 cup blueberries, frozen
- 1 frozen banana cup
- 1 tbsp cooked quinoa
- ½ cup orange juice

Preparation:
1. Blend the frozen bananas and blueberries with a spoon of cooked quinoa in a blender.
2. Add ½ cup orange juice to the mix and blend until smooth and the desired smoothie texture is achieved!
3. Serve in a glass with some garnish as desired.

22. Cleansing Smoothie with Berries for Kidneys

Ingredients:
- ¾ up unsweetened almond milk
- 1 cup fresh or frozen strawberries
- ¾ cup blueberries, frozen

Preparation:
1. If you're using fresh strawberries, wash them beforehand.

2. Fill your blender jar halfway with everything.
3. Blend the mix for 30 to 45 seconds, or until a homogeneous consistency is achieved.

23. Delightful Berry Grape Smoothie

Ingredients:
- 1 cup filtered plain water
- strawberries 34 cup
- ¾ cup pineapple chunks, frozen
- ¼ cup seedless red grapes

Instructions:
1. Strawberries and grapes should be washed.
2. Fill your blender jar halfway with everything.
3. Mix for approximately one minute, or until everything is blended together.

24. Smoothie with Arugula and Greens

Ingredients:
- 1 cup of water
- 1 cup fresh arugula
- 1 cup pineapple chunks, frozen
- ½ cup fresh or frozen strawberries

- 1 apple

Instructions:
1. The arugula leaves should be washed.
2. If using fresh strawberries, wash them first.
3. The apple should be washed, cored, and chopped.
4. Fill your blender jar halfway with everything.
5. Depending on the power of your blender, mix for 60-90 seconds.

25. Smoothie with Strawberries and Pineapple

Ingredients:
¾ cup purified water
1 cup fresh strawberries
1 cup pineapple chunks, frozen

Instructions:
1. Strawberries should be washed.
2. Fill your blender jar halfway with everything.
3. Blend the mix for 30 to 45 seconds, or until a homogeneous consistency is achieved.

26. Blueberry Banana Peanut Smoothie with Low Protein

Ingredients:
- 100 g frozen wild blueberries (equivalent to a heaping half cup)
- 75 g frozen spinach (about a heaping half cup)
- 1 large banana
- 3 tablespoons unrefined peanut oil
- 2 tsp erythritol monk fruit sweetener
- 1 teaspoon vanilla extract
- 8 to 10 oz. cold water

Preparation:
1. Blend all of the ingredients in a blender on high until smooth.
2. Serve and have fun!

Nutritional information:
- 495 calories, 3.4g protein, 35g carbohydrates, 8g fiber, 15g sugar, 41g fat, 66mg sodium, 544mg potassium, 63mg phosphorus, 124mg calcium

27. Blueberry Smoothie with Low Potassium

Ingredients:

- A quarter cup of frozen blueberries
- 1-quart rice milk
- 1 tsp honey or sugar replacement, such as Stevia
- 1 fresh mint sprig
- Optional ice cubes depending on desired thickness
- Protein powder and/or unflavored fiber are optional (but would be great additions).

Instructions:

1. In a blender, combine the blueberries, rice milk, honey, mint, and additional ice (if using).
2. Pour the contents into a big glass, drink and enjoy.

Nutritional information:

- Calories: 142kcal | Carbohydrates: 31g | Protein: 1g | Fat: 2g | Saturated Fat: 1g | Polyunsaturated Fat: 1g | Monounsaturated Fat: 1g | Sodium: 93mg | Potassium: 34mg | Fiber: 1g | Sugar: 15g | Vitamin A: 62IU

28. Smoothie with Blueberries Blast

Ingredients:

- 1 cup blueberries, frozen
- 8 Splenda® packets

- 6 teaspoons protein powder
- 8 cubes of ice
- 14 oz. apple juice (no sugar added)

Preparation:

- Mix all the ingredients in a blender until they are blended together smoothly.

Nutritional information:

- 108 calories, 9g protein, 18g carbohydrates, 0g fat, 0mg cholesterol, 27mg sodium, 183mg potassium, 42mg phosphorus, 57mg calcium, 1.2g fiber.

29. Smoothie with Pineapple and Protein

Ingredients:

- ¾ cup sherbet or sorbet pineapple
- 1 sprinkling of vanilla whey protein powder
- 1 cup of water
- 2 ice cubes, if desired

Preparation:

1. Blend pineapple sherbet, whey protein powder, and water in a blender (ice cubes optional).
2. Blend for 30 to 45 seconds right away.

Tip:

- To make the smoothie thicker, add one or two ice cubes. If you like a milkshake consistency, add one extra ice cube or place it in the freezer for five minutes before serving.

Nutritional info:

- Calories: 268; Protein: 18g; Carbohydrates: 40g; Fat: 4g; Cholesterol: 36mg; Sodium: 93mg; Potassium: 237mg; Phosphorus: 160mg; Calcium: 160mg; Fiber: 1.4g

30. Fruity Smoothie

Ingredients:

- 8 oz. canned fruit cocktail, juiced
- 2 scoops whey protein powder with vanilla flavor
- 1 cup iced water
- 1 pound crushed ice

Preparation:

1. Put all the ingredients in a blender and mix them together.
2. Divide into two servings and serve.

Nutritional info:

- Calories: 186; Protein: 23g; Carbohydrates: 19g; Fat: 2g; Cholesterol: 41mg; Sodium: 62mg; Potassium: 282mg; Phosphorus: 118mg; Calcium: 160mg; Fiber: 1.1g

31. Smoothie with Cucumber Festivus

Ingredients:

- 1 cup cucumber, sliced and peeled
- 1 frozen pineapple cup
- 1 cup celery, sliced
- 1 squeezed lemon.
- Lime, half-squeezed.
- Add ginger to taste

Preparation:

1. Peel and chop the cucumber before adding it to the blender.
2. Cut the celery into pieces and add it to the mix.
3. Squeeze the lemon and lime into the mixer. To taste, add a dash of ginger.
4. Blend until smooth and the ideal smoothie texture is achieved!

32. Green Smoothie for Kidney Care

Ingredients:

- 1 teaspoon (5 g) parsley
- 1 cup cucumber
- 1 tbsp lemon juice

- 1 cup (200 mL) water

Preparation:

1. The first step is to thoroughly wash the parsley. Set it aside as you wash the cucumber. Remove the skin of the cucumber and dice it into small cubes.
2. Squeeze the lemon juice into the blender and whirl.
3. Then combine the other ingredients: parsley, cucumber, and 1 cup water.
4. Blend for a few seconds, then serve in your favorite glass.

33. Cucumber Kidney Cleansing Smoothie

Ingredients:

- ¼ cup of water
- 1 peeled cucumber or 2-3 celery stalks
- 1 apple
- 1 thick (1" X 3") beet slice
- 2 lemons or limes juice (or a combination of the two)
- A pinch of parsley
- 1 tbsp (optional) olive oil

Instructions:

- Combine all of the ingredients. Drink before and after meals.

34. Blend of Green Fever

Ingredients:

- 1 frozen medium banana
- ¼ avocado hass
- 1 huge bunch of spinach
- 2-3 dates
- 1 cup almond milk, unsweetened
- Lime juice squeeze

Preparation:

1. Blend the frozen bananas, avocado, cauliflower, and a handful of spinach in a blender.
2. Remove the seeds from your dates and add them to your mix.
3. Blend in the cup of milk until smooth and the desired smoothie texture is achieved!
4. Serve the smoothie in a glass and enjoy!

35. The Aspirant Blend

Ingredients:

- 1 frozen medium banana (6-8 inches)
- 3 tbsp natural creamy peanut butter
- 1-quart almond milk
- 1 tbsp cocoa powder, unsweetened

- 1 teaspoon Stevia (optional) (for added sweetness)

Preparation:

1. Blend the frozen bananas, almond milk, peanut butter, cocoa butter, and spinach cups in a blender.
2. If preferred, add a cup of almond milk and a spoonful of stevia to the mixture.
3. Blend until smooth and the desired smoothie texture is achieved!
4. Smoothie should be served in a glass.

36. Apple Addiction Smoothie

Ingredients:

- 2-4 OZ. frozen apple sauce cup (no added sugar)
- 1-quart almond milk
- 2 teaspoons toasted oats
- 2 tbsp. almond butter or peanut butter
- ¼ teaspoon cinnamon powder

Preparation:

1. Blend in the frozen apple sauce, oats, peanut butter, or almond butter, and a teaspoon of cinnamon.
2. Blend in the cup of almond milk until smooth and you have the desired smoothie texture!

3. Serve the smoothie in a glass and enjoy!

37. Smoothie With Vitamins and Detox

Ingredients:
- 1 apple
- 1 tablespoon (25 g) honey
- 1 tablespoon (15 g) aloe vera gel
- 1 cup (200 mL) water

Preparation:
1. Select an apple (preferably from an organic orchard). Thoroughly wash the apple, remove the skin, and divide it into four sections.
2. Then comes that spoonful of aloe. Simply cut apart a little portion of the plant and scrape out that tablespoon. It's simple!
3. Simply combine all of the ingredients in a blender and mix until you have a smooth smoothie prepared with apple, honey, aloe, and water.

Tip: Remember to consume this natural smoothie twice a week.

38. Smoothie for Kidney Detoxification

Ingredients:
- 1 cup unsweetened almond milk
- 1 cup fresh arugula
- 1 cup pineapple chunks, frozen
- 1 apple, green

Instructions:
1. Thoroughly wash the arugula leaves.
2. The apple should be washed, cored, and chopped.
3. Fill your blender jar halfway with everything.
4. Blend on high for 60-90 seconds, or until smooth.

39. Papaya Smoothie

Ingredients:
- 3 oz. papaya, sliced into tiny pieces
- ½ cup almond or oat milk, unsweetened
- 1 tablespoon honey
- ½ teaspoon grated fresh ginger
- 2 teaspoons lime juice
- 2 cubes of ice

Instructions:

1. In a blender, combine the papaya, milk, honey, ginger, and lime.
2. Process for 15 seconds at medium speed.
3. Pour in the ice cubes.
4. Process for 30 seconds on high speed to smooth; longer if required.
5. Pour into glasses and serve.

Cooking Hint:

- Peeling ginger to grate can be challenging. Another method is to scrape the skin off with the edge of a teaspoon; the skin will peel right off.

Nutritional Information: Calories: 84, Fat: 2g, Saturated fat: 1g, Trans, Carbohydrates: 18g, Sugar: 13g, Fiber: 2g, Protein: 1g, Sodium: 93 mg, Calcium: 257 mg, Phosphorus: 25 mg, Potassium: 279 mg

40. The Smoothie with Chocolate

Ingredients:

- 2 scoops whey protein with chocolate flavor
- 2 cups of ice
- ½ cup drained evaporated milk
- ¼ cup sweetened condensed milk
- ¼ teaspoon cinnamon powder
- 1 tsp. nutmeg

Preparation:

1. In a blender, combine all ingredients except the cinnamon and process on high for 1-2 minutes, or until smooth.
2. To serve, top with whipped cream and sprinkle with cinnamon.

Nutritional info:

- Calories: 142 calories, Total Fat: 4g, Cholesterol: 18mg, Sodium: 134mg, Carbohydrates: 17g, Protein: 10g, Phosphorus: 162mg, Potassium: 247mg, Dietary Fiber: 0.9g, Calcium: 204mg

41. Smoothies for a Healthy Night's Sleep

Ingredients:

- 1 cup (200 mL) pure coconut water
- ½ cup (100 g) boiled pumpkin flesh
- 1 tablespoon (25 g) honey

Preparation:

1. You can create this drink in five minutes if the pumpkin has previously been cooked or roasted.
2. All you have to do is combine the coconut water, pumpkin, and honey in a blender.

Tip: Blend everything for a few seconds and drink it after supper, two hours before bed.

42. Smoothie Made With Watermelon

Ingredients:
- 4 watermelons (about 125g each)
- 8 ice cubes
- Half a lemon juice

Preparation:
1. Remove the seeds and cut the meat into tiny pieces.
2. Crush the ice cubes coarsely.
3. Place in a blender with the lemon juice and purée.
4. Pour the smoothie into four glasses and serve immediately, since the liquid will rapidly separate.

Tip:
- If your melon isn't extremely sweet, try adding some honey. To add some variation, mix in some mint and basil.

Nutritional info:
- Calories: 60 kcal, fat 0g, sodium 3mg, carbs 13g, protein 1g, phosphorus 15mg, potassium 174mg, liquid 188ml

43. Smoothie With Watermelon And Cucumber

Ingredients:
- 2 cups watermelon, frozen
- One medium cucumber was peeled and cut
- 2 mint sprigs (just the leaves)
- 1 celery stalk
- 1 lime squeeze

Preparation:
1. After peeling the cucumber, slice it up.
2. Cut the celery stalk into squares before placing it in the blender.
3. Blender filled with frozen cucumber and watermelon.
4. Include the two mint springs.
5. Squeeze some lemon juice into your beverage.
6. Blend until the desired smoothie texture is reached.

Nutritional info:
- Calories 143, Fat 0.9g, Carbohydrates 35.2g, Sodium 41.1mg, Protein 4.1g, Potassium 887mg, Phosphorus 115mg, Calcium 85.4mg.

44. Berries with Low Phosphorus

Ingredients:

- ½ cup Vanilla Nepro with Carbohydrate Steady
- ½ cup mixed frozen berries
- 2 tbsp Whipped Nondairy Topping
- Optional: Crystal Light Strawberry Orange Banana
- Water

Instructions:

- Blend all of the ingredients for 45-60 seconds. Add water as needed to get the desired consistency based on your fluid requirements or constraints, as well as your tastes.

Frequently Asked Questions About Healthy Smoothies and Kidney Failure Meals

What Are the Potential Side Effects of Smoothies for Dialysis and CKD Patients?

Consider elements such as caffeine consumption, hydration demands, fruit combinations, juicing advantages, and nutrient balance when assessing the potential adverse effects of drinking smoothies for CKD and dialysis patients.

Caffeine in excess can cause dehydration and worsen symptoms associated with renal disease and dialysis problems.

Furthermore, a dietary imbalance might worsen a patient's health if they do not consume enough protein or other necessary vitamins and minerals.

For these reasons, it's a good idea to check with your doctor before starting any new juice diet or smoothie program.

What other dietary modifications should I make to improve my kidney health?

If you want to improve your kidney health, you need to think about more than simply what you drink.

Eating patterns, salt consumption, activity levels, protein sources, and hydration levels are all important variables in improving or maintaining kidney function. Following a low-salt renal diet becomes simpler with practice.

Begin by reducing your intake of processed foods and added salt, both of which may be unexpectedly high in sodium content. Instead of red meat or certain dairy items, choose leaner proteins like fish and chicken.

Additionally, drink plenty of water throughout the day - eight 8-ounce glasses is a reasonable rule of thumb, although this may vary depending on your stage of kidney disease.

Exercise regularly, even if it's only 15-30 minutes of moderate aerobic physical activity every day. Following these recommendations will go a long way toward keeping your kidneys healthy.

Are there any smoothie recipes that are specifically designed for diabetics?

There are many wonderful taste combinations and alternative components that may be utilized in the recipes to help regulate your sugar levels and support your kidney health. Modifications to recipes may also help make them more suited for diabetics.

From creamy avocado blends to delicious banana mixes with no added sugars, these healthy yet delightful solutions provide much-needed nutrients while fulfilling cravings - something that all diabetics will appreciate!

To reduce the sugar content, just replace any sugar or honey in the recipe with an artificial sweetener.

You may also add additional fibrous vegetables or entire fruits to the mix to enhance the fiber content, which slows carbohydrate digestion and absorption. Other suggestions include substituting water for milk (renal diet milk) or juice in your smoothie.

How Often Should I Drink Smoothies for Healthy Kidneys?

When it comes to nutrition, finding the correct balance of frequency of consumption is critical. Drinking a kidney-friendly smoothie every day, along with a balanced diet, is generally suggested as part of a healthy lifestyle.

The amount and frequency with which you consume smoothies will be determined by a variety of criteria, including your kidney disease stage, weight, age, gender, and other medical problems. To help you find the correct balance for you, consult with a healthcare expert such as your doctor or a nutritionist.

With these tips in mind, you'll be well on your way to enjoying tasty smoothies while maintaining your kidneys in excellent condition.

Is it possible to find smoothie recipes that are suitable for vegetarians and vegans?

To ensure that your kidney health is taken care of when living a vegetarian or vegan lifestyle, use plant-based foods and low-sugar replacements.

Choose dairy-free alternatives such as almond milk or coconut water. Try including fiber-rich alternatives such as chia seeds into any smoothie you make for increased nourishment.

Making vegetarian smoothies is an easy and tasty way to get your daily dosage of fruits and veggies.

To prepare a vegetarian smoothie, combine fresh or frozen fruit with milk, yogurt, or a milk substitute such as almond milk or coconut milk in a blender.

You may also add some protein and healthy fats by adding seeds, nuts, or nut butter. A spoonful of honey or maple syrup can be added for extra sweetness. Blend all of the ingredients and enjoy your smoothie!

To make a standard smoothie vegan, simply replace the milk with a milk substitute, the yogurt with vegan yogurt, and the honey with a vegan sweetener like agave syrup or date syrup.

You may also use protein-rich items like chia seeds, hemp seeds, or protein powder. A typical smoothie recipe may be easily changed into a vegan smoothie recipe with a few easy tweaks.

CONCLUSION

Remember that you are not alone as you begin your renal diet smoothie adventure. Numerous people with renal illness have successfully introduced smoothies into their diets, finding restored vigor and passion for life.

Reflect on your astonishing metamorphosis as you wrap up your culinary excursion. You've adopted a new approach to kidney-conscious eating that feeds your body while still pleasing your taste buds.

Remember that your experience with renal-friendly smoothies is only getting started. Continue to try new dishes, experiment with different ingredients, and relish the tastes that call to you. Each smoothie you make demonstrates your perseverance, ingenuity, and dedication
n to your health.

Remember that you can fuel your body and uplift your soul with tasty and healthy smoothies as you begin each new day. Allow these culinary delights to remind you of your courage and tenacity in the face of renal illness.

To my valued reader,

As you complete my culinary voyage with renal-friendly smoothies, I want to express my deepest thanks for your willingness to join me on this expedition. Your excitement and passion for kidney-friendly food were the driving forces behind the production of this book.

Thank you for embracing the power of food to change your perspective on renal health. May these smoothies feed your bodies, energize your spirits, and encourage you to live a life full of taste and vitality.

FOR OTHER BOOKS WRITTEN BY THE AUTHOR

Scan This 👇